PSORIASIS

Treating and Managing Psoriasis

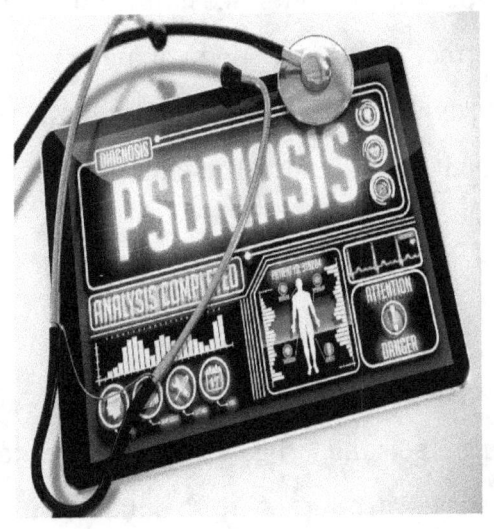

By

Paolo Jose de Luna

Paolo Jose De Luna

This document is geared towards providing exact and reliable information in regards to the topic and issue covered. The publication is sold with the idea that the publisher is not required to render accounting, officially permitted, or otherwise, qualified services. If advice is necessary, legal or professional, a practiced individual in the profession should be ordered.

In no way is it legal to reproduce, duplicate, or transmit any part of this document in either electronic means or in printed format. Recording of this publication is strictly prohibited and any storage of this document is not allowed unless with

Paolo Jose De Luna

The information herein is offered for informational purposes solely, and is universal as so. The presentation of the information is without contract or any type of guarantee assurance.

The trademarks that are used are without any consent, and the publication of the trademark is without permission or backing by the trademark owner. All trademarks and brands within this book are for clarifying purposes only and are the owned by the owners themselves, not affiliated with this document.

Table of Contents

INTRODUCTION

The skin is considered to be the biggest organ in the body, covering about 80% of the total body surface. This means that the skin is easily exposed since it covers most of the body, making it the first thing anyone would see when they interact with other people. Using our visual abilities, the skin is easily seen and this makes the skin quite important. The horrors of skin disease often plague a lot of people and even more dread the thought of having scars, lesions, and wounds on the skin. With the various bacteria and viruses going around, you can never tell what kind of illness that can affect you – including your skin. One of the most well-recognized skin diseases is psoriasis which is often considered as troublesome and dreadful by a lot of people.

Psoriasis is a skin condition that often leads to the appearance of plaques on the skin, making it look flaky and scaly. These dry flakes located on the skin can cause scaling and are speculated to be caused by the abnormally fast proliferation of the skin cells due to the inflammatory response of the specialized WBCs or white blood cells known as "lymphocytes". This skin disease often affects areas like the scalp, the elbows, and the knees, but it can also affect other areas such as the nape and the back.

The severity of psoriasis can vary, ranging from mild up to severe. Psoriasis can be as minor as they may not even be detected by the person who has it or it can also be severe that it can cover the entirety of a person's skin, leading to low self-esteem and a huge hit on someone's self-confidence since the skin is the first thing that anyone sees in a person.

Psoriasis is found to be an incurable and chronic skin disease. While it has a variable course, psoriasis can either improve or worsen, depending on the interventions and the measures used to manage it. It's not surprising that psoriasis can remain dormant for years or even stay in remission for many years. However, there are also those people who have reported the worsening of psoriasis due to a number of factors like the change in weather conditions, especially during the winter season.

Psoriasis

While it may be a dreadful disease for many people, psoriasis is by no means contagious and there are a number of ways that you can employ to decrease your risk of developing this skin disorder. Aside from that, thorough management of the skin disease can also ensure a good outlook on the severity of psoriasis by following the medication regimen prescribed by your physician, eating a balanced diet, staying away from risk factors that increase the likelihood of developing psoriasis, and a whole lot more.

In this book, you'll be learning everything about the skin disease -Psoriasis and how to deal with it. This would include details about psoriasis, the signs and symptoms of this disease, the number of diagnostic tests available to detect psoriasis, and how to manage psoriasis using medical intervention and even using a number of home remedies to treat this skin disease.

Chapter 1 - What is Psoriasis?

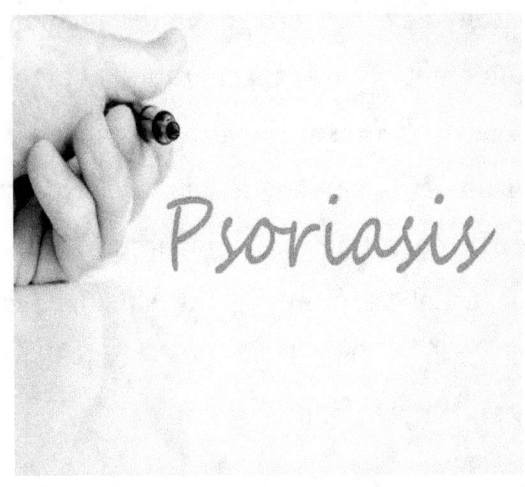

Psoriasis is a skin condition that is often described as a chronic skin disease that is characterized by the formation of plaques and dry flakes which results in the skin looking scaly and flaky. Years of extensive study has proven that one of the main causes of psoriasis is the body's abnormal response to the inflammatory reaction in the skin which is controlled by the white blood cells called the "lymphocytes". These white blood cells are designed to fight off infection and other foreign matter and help in the repair and regeneration of the tissues. In the case of psoriasis, however, the skin ends up having an abnormally faster regeneration rate compared to what is the usual, resulting in the skin having raised lesions that is often described as scaly and unpleasant to look at.

Due to the accelerated healing mechanism of the skin, the newer skin cells actually move upwards to the skin surface in just a couple of days instead of the usual weeks. This results in the appearance of patches on the skin as raised plaques. These patches can either be mild to severe, affecting various areas like the elbows, the knees, and the scalp. However, other areas can also be affected by psoriasis like the back, the nape, the hands, and the feet. In terms of prevalence, psoriasis is found to be more common in adults, but it can also affect children, teenagers, and the elderly.

Psoriasis has a wide reach and can affect all races and for both male and female. Though psoriasis can affect people from various age groups, it is primarily more common among those in the early adulthood years of their life. The overall quality of life is the first thing that takes a hit when a person is diagnosed with psoriasis because of its effect on the person's outward appearance. It is only recently that studies have shown that those with psoriasis are more prone to develop other health problems like diabetes mellitus, hyperlipidemia, increased blood pressure, atherosclerosis, myocardial infarction, and other cardiovascular diseases in the future. This can be correlated as to how inflammation has a major role in psoriasis and also among these health problems. In order to treat psoriasis, a strong and committed healthcare team is necessary to provide the best type of care for a person diagnosed with psoriasis.

In some cases, psoriasis can also affect the nails which leads to the separation of the nails and the nailbeds. Another complication that may arise because of psoriasis is a condition known as psoriatic arthritis which is a form of arthritis arising from psoriasis that primarily affects the joints which is more common among the elderly.

Causes and Risk Factors of Psoriasis

While the exact cause of psoriasis is still unknown, there are a number of factors that increase the risk of developing psoriasis. Genetic predisposition and a number of environmental factors may increase the likelihood of psoriasis, but those are still dependent for each individual. Studies have shown that psoriasis has a tendency to run in the family, but it doesn't necessarily mean that if you have a family member has psoriasis, you will definitely develop psoriasis in the future.

Research has also shown that the immune system plays an important role in the case of psoriasis since psoriasis is thought to be dependent on the body's response to foreign matter or infection.

However, even through extensive research and studies, the exact cause of psoriasis that triggers it in the first place still remains to be a mystery in the healthcare industry. Though there may have been speculations about the triggering mechanism of psoriasis, there is still not enough scientific evidence to prove these hypotheses.

The Different Types of Psoriasis

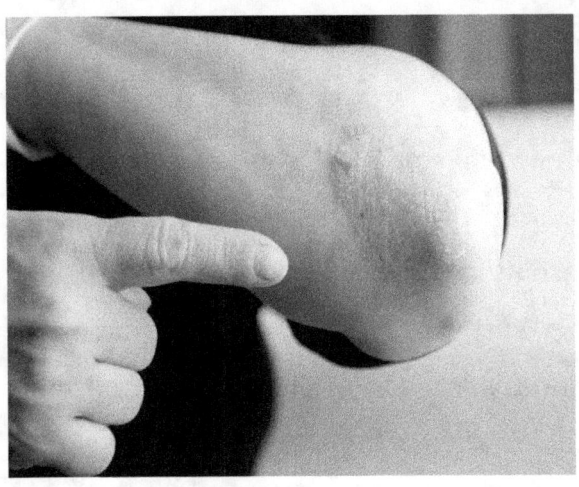

As a skin disease, psoriasis can be classified into several different types depending on the area that it affects and the characteristics of the skin changes that occur. Here are the following types of psoriasis:

- Psoriasis Vulgaris – the most common type of psoriasis and appears in the form of plaque-like formations on the skin.

- Guttate Psoriasis – this type of psoriasis forms small and drop-like spots on the skin.

- Inverse Psoriasis – as its name implies, inverse psoriasis grows in the folds of the skin which can be found on the navel, the buttocks, the underarms, and more.

- Pustular Psoriasis – this type of psoriasis leads to the formation of blisters that are filled with pus.

- Palmoplantar Psoriasis – a type of psoriasis that primarily affects the palms and the soles.

- Erythodermic Psoriasis – this type of psoriasis covers the entire surface of the skin, characterized by a reddish discoloration of the skin and it can lead to the skin being cold and it may even lead to congestive heart failure.

Psoriasis

- Nail psoriasis – a type of psoriasis that is characterized by yellow-pitted nails and can lead to the separation of the nail from the nailbed; often considered to be difficult to treat, treatment of nail psoriasis involves the use of strong topical steroids that are applied on the affected nailbed and even injecting steroids on the nailbed of the cuticle.

- Scalp psoriasis – severe cases of this type of psoriasis is known to lead to hair loss, excessive dandruff, and itchiness of the scalp.

Signs and Symptoms of Psoriasis

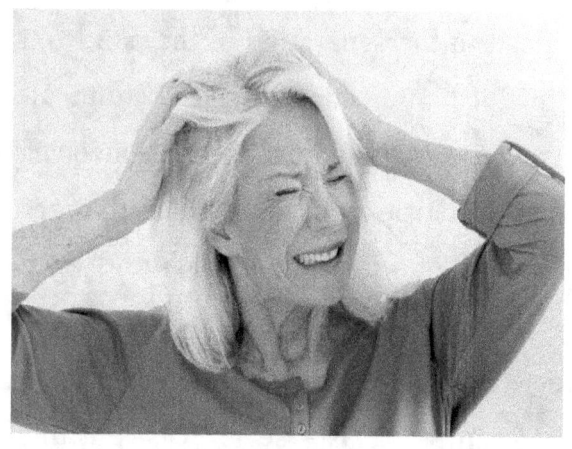

The signs and symptoms of psoriasis mainly focuses on the affected area of the skin. With the various types of psoriasis, assessing the signs and symptoms is important to establish a concrete diagnosis of psoriasis. What makes psoriasis so difficult to treat is because of its identification since it can be easily mistaken as a fungal skin infection. Most often, psoriasis affects areas like the elbows, the scalp, and the knees, but it can also affect other areas as well. Here are the signs and symptoms that you should watch out for to identify psoriasis:

- Reddish or pinkish scaly bumps on the skin
- Plaque formation on the skin
- Itchiness
- Auzpitz sign – a medical diagnostic sign for psoriasis characterized by a blood spot on the skin when you pull off a part of the scaly skin in areas affected by psoriasis
- Pinpoint depressions of the fingernails and toenails
- Distal Onycholysis – yellowish to brown separations that develop between the nails and the nailbeds
- Sore throat – often appears before the development of guttate psoriasis

- Genital lesions – often appears in inverse psoriasis
- Flat red plaques on the skin
- Small bumps filled with pus on the affected area
- Fever and chills
- Brittle fingernails and toenails
- Severe dandruff – often in scalp psoriasis

Chapter 2 - Treatment and Management of Psoriasis

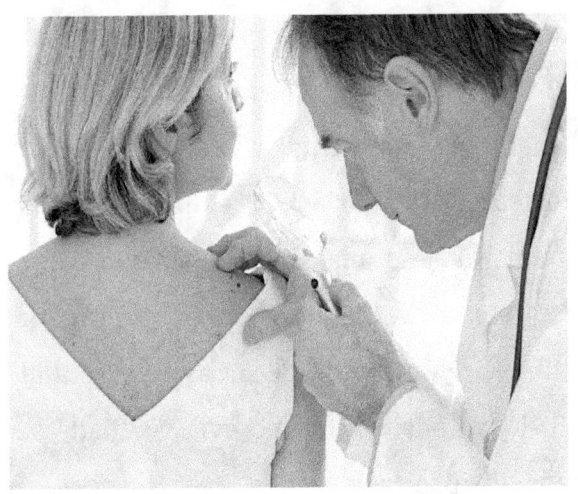

After knowing more about psoriasis, it's time to know on how to deal with it from a medical perspective. There are various treatment options available to use when it comes to managing psoriasis. These include the administration of medications and utilizing preventive measures to decrease the severity and risk of psoriasis from developing in the first place.

Since psoriasis has many different types, you can expect that the treatment options available will be plenty. The different areas affected by psoriasis require various treatments and may not be effective for everyone. Choosing the right treatment option for you should be set as an essential priority to ensure that no delay is made in managing psoriasis.

You have to know first is that psoriasis is *not* contagious. The common misconception of a lot of people is whenever they see a form of skin infection or alteration, they immediately brand it as highly infectious. But that's not the case of psoriasis.

However, psoriasis can complicate into psoriatic arthritis if not treated in time.

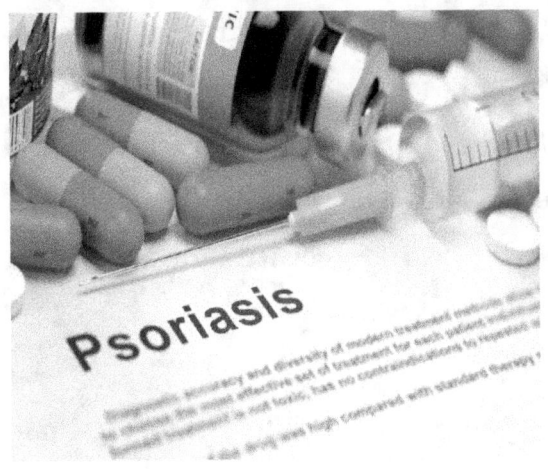

Psoriasis is a complex autoimmune disorder where the body attacks its own skin cells, producing an excessive regeneration process which results in the piling up or stacking of the skin together. The best way to treat psoriasis is to go to a physician and have it diagnosed and treated specifically. Here are the treatment options that you can do in order to treat psoriasis:

• The most common treatment option used for psoriasis is by applying creams, lotions, and other topical solutions to the affected areas of the skin which contain salicylic acid or corticosteroids to help control psoriasis.

• Topical ointments which contain Vitamin D and retinoids are also known to help control the signs and symptoms of psoriasis by applying it to the affected area.

• Application of ultraviolet rays have been shown to be somewhat effective as multiple studies have shown when it comes to resolving the abnormal skin regeneration process in psoriasis.

Psoriasis

• Taking corticosteroids either in oral or as injections can help control the signs and symptoms of psoriasis by acting against the inflammatory response that the body makes in this skin condition.

• Using medicated soaps and lotions are also known to help in keeping the signs and symptoms of psoriasis controlled and limit the further spread of the skin disease.

• Using medicated shampoo for those with scalp psoriasis is found to be effective, relieving the itchiness that psoriasis brings, as well as controlling the excessive dandruff that occurs in scalp psoriasis.

• Toxicity to medications is quite common for chronic conditions like psoriasis, so doctors have suggested to make use of a rotational therapy which is changing the medications used by those with psoriasis after a set amount of time, for example, after 12 to 24 months of taking one medication, the patient should then change to another drug.

• Topical sprays that contain corticosteroids like hydrocortisone can also be applied on the affected areas of the skin to limit the spread of psoriasis; however, using corticosteroid sprays, creams, lotions, or oils too much that exceed the usual dosage and frequency is not advised since it can thin out the skin and cause damage and flaking.

• Calcitriol cream is another useful treatment option for psoriasis because of its action on the calcium metabolism of the body which helps control the spread of the signs and symptoms of psoriasis; today, a combination with topical steroids and calcitriol is quite useful in controlling the affected areas of psoriasis.

• Moisturizers with salicylic acid and glycolic acid help in reducing the scale formation in psoriasis, as well as promoting the adequate hydration of the skin and limiting the dry flaking that is widely recognized in psoriasis.

• Immunomodulators are also considered to be helpful in mild cases of psoriasis by controlling the signs and symptoms of the skin disorder without thinning out the skin; however, a controversy has popped up for discussion whether these immunomodulators should be used as they have been found to have adverse reactions like skin infections and even increasing the risk for cancer.

• Coal tar is another option to provide help in treating psoriasis as this ingredient can help control the appearance of the affected skin areas and even limit the dry flakiness in psoriasis without thinning out the skin.

• Anthralin is an active ingredient that can be found in many creams, lotions, and ointments which can help control the signs and symptoms of psoriasis, effectively limiting its spread, appearance, and flaking; however, it is also known to cause skin irritation and redness in some cases.

Psoriasis

• Application of fish oil directly on the affected areas of psoriasis is said to be helpful as it limits the appearance and the dryness of the skin.

• Acitretin is a drug that can be used to treat a variety of types of psoriasis, but it isn't effective in all types; it can be used by both males and females who are not pregnant or for those who are not planning to be pregnant for three to four years; common side effects of this medication include dry skin, dry eyes, increased levels of cholesterol, and an elevated triglyceride levels in the blood.

• Cyclosporine is another drug that is used to suppress the immune system and prevent the further spread of psoriasis and is also known to be used in treating widespread and complicated cases of psoriasis.

• Methotrexate is often used in rheumatoid arthritis, but it is also known to help treat psoriasis as well, and because of its action, it is quite helpful in treating cases of complications that lead to psoriatic arthritis.

While there are a variety of treatment options available for controlling and managing psoriasis, there is no such thing as a perfect cure. Unfortunately, not everything on this list might work for everyone, but you shouldn't lose hope and get discouraged. While one treatment option may not work for you, others may work instead. What's important is that you should first consult your attending physician regarding these treatments especially since medications may have certain side effects that may counteract with other medical problems that you may be experiencing. Always consult your doctor and always ask the help of a professional when it comes to seeking treatment for psoriasis.

Chapter 3 - Managing Psoriasis at Home

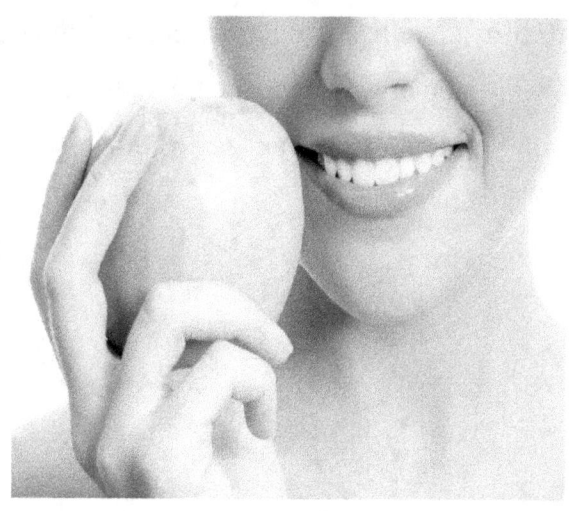

There are a number of medical interventions that can be done to control the signs and symptoms of psoriasis. Since it's a chronic disorder without a specific cure, there is only hope in controlling the skin condition known as psoriasis. Fortunately, many of those who have this condition experience remission periods, some of which have long-lasting remissions that can go on for many years. When it comes to managing psoriasis, it's not just about using various medication or going to the hospital. There are also a variety of home remedies and treatments that you can use to manage psoriasis at home. There are also ways that you can do to reduce the risk of psoriasis from even developing. Here are some of them and you better take note!

• Eat a balanced diet. Nutrients and vitamins like iron, vitamin D, and oils help in reducing the risk of developing psoriasis by promoting a healthy growth and regeneration of the skin.

• Choose soaps, lotions, and other cosmetic products that are labeled as "skin sensitive" as these products help mitigate the damage done to the skin which can lead to the excessive regeneration process that may lead to psoriasis.

• Limit eating red meats and fatty foods as these have been found to increase the risk in getting psoriasis.

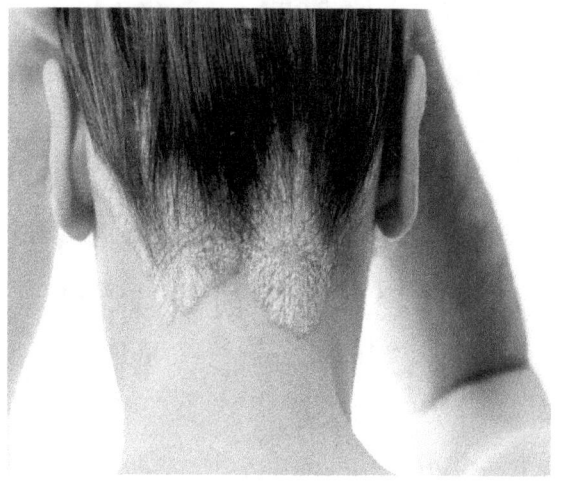

• You can apply olive oil or vegetable oil to the affected areas of the skin to lock in the moisture and contain the nutrients and minerals in the skin, preventing the overgrowth of the psoriatic tissues. Massaging vegetable oil or olive oil on your scalp can also help those with scalp psoriasis.

• Observing proper hygiene and cleanliness is one of the most secure ways that you can prevent the occurrence of psoriasis or even most of the skin disorders that you know about. Having a clean skin will help prevent skin infections and prevent the proliferation of bacteria and viruses that can cause terrible skin conditions.

• Make use of a lukewarm bath together with therapeutic bath salts or soaps which help in promoting the moisture in the skin and removing the dry flaking areas in the affected areas of psoriasis.

- Prevent injuries occurring on the skin as trauma can contribute to the development of psoriasis since psoriasis patches can form almost anywhere on the skin, especially areas that have been previously injured or damaged.

- Reduce stress and anxiety by engaging in a variety of relaxation techniques like deep breathing, yoga, therapeutic massages, and more as stress and anxiety may contribute to the flaring of psoriasis signs and symptoms.

- If you have an infection like a sore throat, better consult your doctor to have it treated quickly as psoriasis can appear in some cases of infection.

- Consult your doctor before taking other medications since some drugs can contribute to the development of psoriasis which may include NSAIDs (Non-Steroidal Anti-Inflammatory Drugs), lithium-containing drugs, and beta-blockers (e.g. metoprolol, bisoprolol, atenolol, etc.).

• Make use of lotions and moisturizers as psoriasis tends to dry up the skin and cause flakiness in some areas, resulting in patches and unpleasant plaques on the skin.

• Don't stay out under the sun for too long as overexposure to sunlight can contribute to the development of psoriasis. In fact, sunlight and heat can exacerbate the signs and symptoms of psoriasis, often producing flares if you're not careful about your time under the sun.

• Avoid drinking alcoholic beverages or smoking cigarettes as studies have found out that these vices contribute to the worsening of psoriasis and even contribute to the development of signs and symptoms of psoriasis.

• Maintain a healthy weight to make sure as exercise and proper diet are still important components when it comes to preventing psoriasis.

Let's face it – not every type of treatment works with everyone. There are a number of ways that you can manage psoriasis at home, but there's no assurance that all of these measures will work for you. In regard to this, it's still your responsibility to keep an eye out for factors that may contribute to the development of psoriasis and instituting measures so that you can prevent psoriasis from occurring in the first place.

A number of studies have shown that there are more possibilities when it comes to managing psoriasis. Some have said that certain food supplements, vitamins, minerals, and more can help limit the signs and symptoms of psoriasis – some even claiming that they do indeed work.

But in all seriousness, the treatment and management of psoriasis is still important and you should always first consult your doctor when it comes to using these home remedies for psoriasis. Aside from these remedies that have been mentioned, you've probably heard another one from somewhere and they even claim that they're the best option that you can possible get. Choose one that works best for you and start working with it to control the signs and symptoms of psoriasis.

Chapter 4 - Myths and Facts on Psoriasis

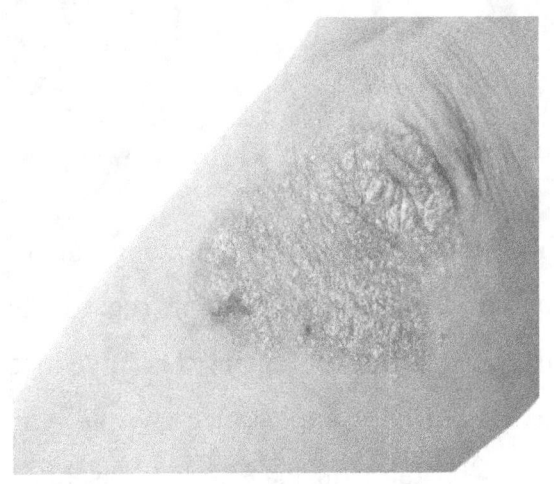

Psoriasis is one of the most recognized and well-known skin conditions in the world. As a healthcare problem, psoriasis has a variety of treatment options in order to manage and control the signs and symptoms of this skin condition. Before judging the condition and someone who has psoriasis, you first need to clear up some misconceptions and misunderstandings about psoriasis to shed more light on this skin disease. Here are some myths and facts that you need to know about psoriasis.

Psoriasis is NOT Contagious

What most people get wrong about psoriasis is that a lot of them regard the skin disease as contagious or infectious because of its appearance. While the plaques on the skin may be unpleasant to look at for the person with psoriasis, there's no evidence that psoriasis can be spread through contact, airborne, or vectors. A lot of people with psoriasis get the judgmental eye of the public because of the outward appearance of the skin, but you should be aware that psoriasis cannot be contracted through any sort of transmission as it often appears out of heredity in the family or out of several factors that may increase the risk of developing psoriasis.

Psoriasis is NOT Curable

Another common misconception about psoriasis is that most people think that there is a cure for the skin condition. Unfortunately, there is no definitive cure for psoriasis. There is no single solution that can block off or stop psoriasis from completely occurring. Psoriasis is a chronic condition that lasts for your whole life. However, there are ways on how you can treat, control, and manage psoriasis which leads us to another common misunderstanding about this skin condition.

Psoriasis is Treatable

While psoriasis is not curable, it is highly treatable. As a chronic condition, if you have psoriasis that would mean you will have it for life. There is no known cure for psoriasis and there is no single solution to halt the signs and symptoms completely. Fortunately, there are various ways that you can do to control the signs and symptoms of psoriasis ranging from medical interventions, administration of medications, home remedies, and alternative treatments. While not everything might not work for one person, some of them may work for you. All you have to do is try and work together with your attending physician to get the best results out of your treatment.

Psoriasis is More Than a Skin Condition

Most people think about psoriasis as a mere skin condition that's just unpleasant to look at. However, that should not be the case as psoriasis is a serious medical condition that involves both the physical and emotional aspects of care for the person. Because of the change in one's outward appearance, the person suffers from discrimination and from the judgmental eyes of society. But psoriasis should be considered as a medical problem just like diabetes mellitus, hypertension, and cardiovascular problems since there are certain complications that can pose risk to one's health like psoriatic arthritis.

Psoriasis is Long-Term

You should know and accept that psoriasis is a condition that is long-term and chronic. That means it just doesn't last for a couple of days or weeks. It can last for years. However, it's a good thing to also know that psoriasis doesn't appear forever. There are periods of remissions that are often experienced by those afflicted with this skin problem through the use of various treatment options, home remedies, and changes in lifestyle to ensure that the development of psoriasis ceases and the signs and symptoms are adequately controlled for the time being.

It's NOT a Rare Disease

While it may look unpleasant and new to the eyes of the masses, psoriasis is far from being a rare skin disease. In fact, psoriasis is quite common around the world with 2% to 5% of people around the world being diagnosed with this condition. That would mean tens of thousands or maybe even millions suffering from psoriasis. It's also considered as one of the most well-known skin conditions around the world due to its easy to recognize signs and symptoms.

Both Men and Women Can Get Psoriasis

There's no gender difference when it comes to getting psoriasis. It doesn't matter if you're a male or female – you still have a chance of getting psoriasis. What matters is that the several factors that can lead to the development of psoriasis should be kept under control so you don't experience the signs and symptoms of this skin disease. Factors like the environment, smoking, drinking alcoholic beverages, eating an unhealthy diet, and the like play crucial factors in psoriasis, as well as other health problems.

Psoriasis is NOT Because of Poor Hygiene

While hygiene may play a role in reducing the risk of developing psoriasis, there is no evidence that tells us that poor hygiene can directly cause psoriasis. Psoriasis appears on the skin, but that doesn't mean that poor hygiene is a direct cause of the skin disorder. The problem lies in the body's immune system wherein it recognizes its own cells as the enemy and reacts by promoting the excessive regeneration of the skin cells, resulting the in the formation of plaques on the skin and thus the appearance of psoriasis.

Psoriasis is NOT Easy to Diagnose

Contrary to popular belief, psoriasis is quite difficult to diagnose. Establishing a strong diagnosis is made difficult because of the vague signs and symptoms of psoriasis, making it hard for anyone to distinguish it from other skin disorders. Skin rashes are quite common as with the appearance of psoriasis on the skin. In fact, other skin conditions may mimic psoriasis like skin allergies brought about by food or medications, eczema, skin infection, and skin irritation. Ruling out other skin conditions is important so that psoriasis is adequately diagnosed and the right treatment options are started immediately.

Wrong Information on Psoriasis is Harmful

Feeding the wrong information about psoriasis can bring more harm that the disease itself. Spread misinformation among the masses about psoriasis is a serious issue and it needs to be stopped. You should first research and study about psoriasis before you feed others this information. It not only affects those who have psoriasis but is also affects the outlook of those around them. It severely cripples the self-esteem of those with psoriasis because of their outer appearance and giving wrong information to people, especially about common myths and misconceptions about psoriasis, should be stopped once and for all.

There are certainly a lot more misconceptions and misunderstandings about psoriasis. Of course, there's no quick way on changing the beliefs of the people and psoriasis is no exception to that rule. But learning information about psoriasis is the first step that should be taken when it comes to educating the public. As they say, you need to first educate yourself before you can start thinking about teaching others. Learn more about psoriasis and wash away the discrimination towards those afflicted by this skin problem.

CONCLUSION

Psoriasis is one of the most common skin conditions worldwide. It's widely recognized and is known as a health problem that should be treated with medical interventions. It starts out as a plaque formation on the skin due to the excessive regeneration of the skin cells due to the damage that occurs on the skin because of a problem in the immune system.

However, psoriasis is a chronic skin problem that has no definitive cure. There's no stopping it and there's no way that you can cure it completely. But *is* highly treatable with the variety of treatment options with medications, home remedies, and alternative treatments available to utilize.

Before you start dreading psoriasis, know that there are ways on how you can control the signs and symptoms of psoriasis. The first step should be clearing up the misconceptions of this skin condition and be enlightened more about this skin disease.